The ultimate lean and green diet cookbook

Delicious and tasty seafood recipes to weight loss

Lisa Reims

Table of contents

Seafood recipes

Mustard Salmon With Herbs 7

Nutty Coconut Fish 9

Olive Oil Poached Tuna 11

One-Pot Tuna Casserole 13

Bacon-Wrapped Salmon 15

Bagna Cauda 17

Bermuda Fish Chowder 18

Salmon Tikka 21

Almond And Parmesan Crusted Tilapia 22

Crab And Shrimp Pasta Salad 25

Cream Of Salmon Soup 27

Creamed Salmon On Toast 30

Coconut Salsa on Chipotle Fish Tacos 33

Baked Cod Crusted with Herbs 35

Cajun Garlic Shrimp Noodle Bowl 37

Crazy Saganaki Shrimp 39

Creamy Bacon-Fish Chowder 41

Crisped Coco-Shrimp with Mango Dip................................ 43

Cucumber-Basil Salsa on Halibut Pouches 45

Salmon with Mustard.. 48

Dijon Mustard and Lime Marinated Shrimp....................... 51

Dill Relish on White Sea Bass 53

Salmon & Arugula Omelet 55

Tuna Omelet..57

Fish Stew 59

Salmon & Veggie Salad.. 61

Tuna Salad... 62

Shrimp & Greens Salad 65

Shrimp, Apple & Carrot Salad...67

Shrimp & Green Beans Salad 69

Shrimp & Olives Salad... 71

Shrimp & Arugula Salad...73

Shrimp & Veggies Salad 74

Salmon Lettuce Wraps 77

Tuna Burgers 78

Spicy Salmon 81

Lemony Salmon.. 83

Zesty Salmon 85

Stuffed Salmon 87

Salmon with Asparagus 89

Salmon Parcel 91

Salmon with Cauliflower Mash 93

Salmon with Salsa 95

Walnut Crusted Salmon 97

Garlicky Tilapia 99

Tilapia Piccata 100

Cod in Dill Sauce 103

Cod & Veggies Bake 105

Cod & Veggie Pizza 107

Garlicky Haddock 109

Mustard Salmon With Herbs

Prep time: 10 min

Cook Time: 30 min

Serving: 2

Ingredients:

- mustard
- mayonnaise
- dressing mix
- garlic powder, or to taste
- lemons
- salmon fillet
- 1 sprig fresh mint, stemmed, or to taste
- 1 sprig fresh rosemary, or to taste
- 2 spoons chopped fresh chives, or to taste
- 1 sprig fresh dill, or to taste
- 4 cloves garlic, crushed, or to taste

Instructions:

1.In a bowl, combine garlic powder, ranch dressing, Italian dressing, mayonnaise, and mustard. Squeeze over the mixture with 1/2 of the lemon. Cut the leftover lemon halves

2.Put the preheated oven in and cook for 30-45 minutes before the flesh can easily flake with a fork.

Nutrition: Calories 277, Fat 11, Carbs 26, Protein 18, Sodium 520

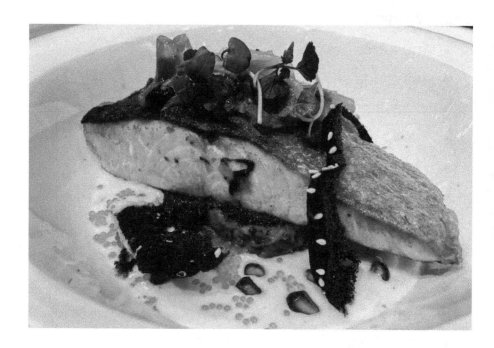

Nutty Coconut Fish

Prep time: 10 min

Cook Time: 30 min

Serving: 2

Ingredients:

- mayonnaise
- mustard
- bread crumbs
- shredded coconut
- mixed nuts
- granulated sugar
- 1 teaspoon salt
- 1/2 teaspoon cayenne pepper
- 1 pound whitefish fillets

Instructions:

1.The oven should be preheated to 190-195 degrees C.

2.Blend brown mustard and mayonnaise in a small bowl. Mix cayenne pepper, salt, sugar, chopped mixed nuts, shredded coconut, and dry breadcrumbs in a medium bowl.

3.Dip fish in mayonnaise mixture, then dip in breadcrumb mixture. In a baking dish, put coated fish fillets.

4.Bake for 20/3 minutes in a preheated oven until the fish flakes easily with a fork.

Nutrition: Calories 180, Fat 2, Carbs 12, Protein 6, Sodium 426

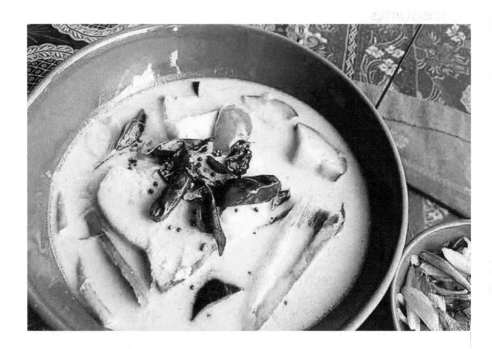

Olive Oil Poached Tuna

Prep time: 10 min

Cook Time: 30 min

Serving: 2

Ingredients:

- tuna steaks
- garlic
- thyme
- pepper flakes
- olive oil
- sea salt to taste

Instructions:

1.Set aside tuna for 10-15 minutes at room temperature.

2.In a heavy pan, mix red pepper flakes, garlic, and thyme. Pour in olive oil until an inch deep. On medium heat, heat for 5-10 minutes until the thyme and garlic sizzles.

3.Put the tuna lightly in the pan of hot oil, then turn heat to low. Cook steaks for 5-7 minutes while constantly spooning oil on top until the tuna is hot and white. Take off heat, move the steaks to a baking pan, and then pour hot oil and herbs on top. Let the fish cool down to temperature.

4.Use plastic wrap to tightly cover the baking dish and put the steaks in the refrigerator for 24 hours. Take the tuna out of the oil and top with sea salt.

Nutrition: Calories 208, Fat 21, Carbs 26, Protein 36, Sodium 543

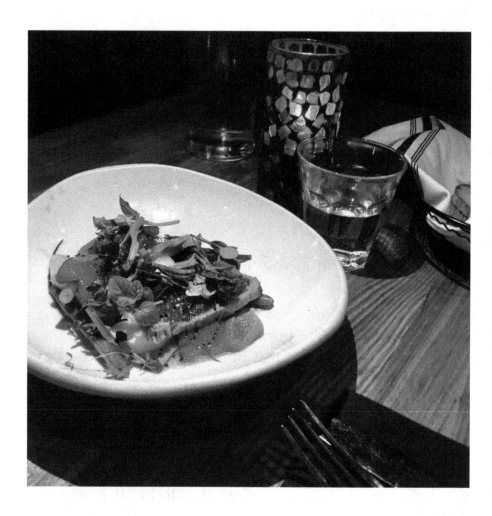

One-Pot Tuna Casserole

Prep time: 10 min

Cook Time: 20 min

Serving: 2

Ingredients:

- 1 (16 ounces) package egg noodles
- 1 (10 ounces) package frozen green peas, thawed
- 1/4 cup butter
- 1 (10.75 ounces) can condense cream of mushroom soup
- 1 (5 ounces) can tuna, drained
- 1/4 cup milk
- 1 cup shredded Cheddar cheese

Instructions:

1.Boil a big pot with lightly salted water. Cook pasta in boiling water, till "al dente"; add peas at 3 final minutes of cooking and drain.

2.Melt butter overheats in the same pot. Add Cheddar cheese, milk, tuna, and mushroom soup; mix till mixture is smooth and cheese melts. Mix peas and pasta in till evenly coated.

Nutrition: Calories 398, Fat 16, Carbs 12, Protein 33, Sodium 455

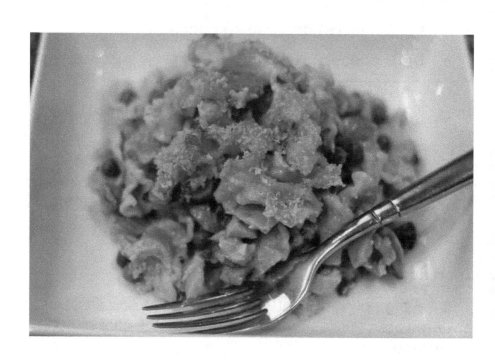

Bacon-Wrapped Salmon

Prep time: 10 min

Cook Time: 30 min

Serving: 2

Ingredients:

- 4 (4 ounces) skin-on salmon fillets
- 1 teaspoon garlic powder
- 1 teaspoon dried dill weed
- salt and pepper to taste
- 1/2 pound bacon, cut in half

Instructions:

1.Preheat oven to 375°F. Generously brush olive oil on a cookie sheet.

2.Arrange salmon fillets skin down on the cookie sheet. Season fillets with dill, salt, pepper, and garlic powder. Cover the fillets completely with bacon strips. Arrange the bacon so they don't overlap each other.

3.Bake in the oven for 20-23 minutes, just until the fish's center is not translucent. To broil, change the oven setting and cook for another 1 to 2 minutes until the bacon becomes crispy.

Nutrition: Calories 307, Fat 23, Carbs 8, Protein 16, Sodium 590

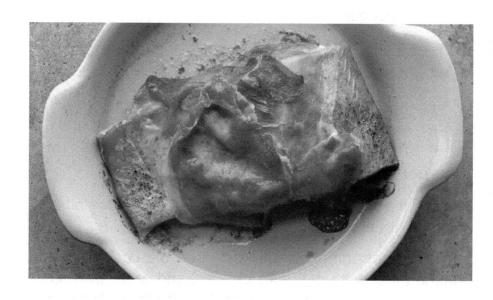

Bagna Cauda

Prep time: 10 min

Cook Time: 30 min

Serving: 2

Ingredients:

- 1/2 cup butter
- 10 cloves garlic, minced
- fillets
- cream

Instructions:

1.Mix in garlic and cook until softened. Lower the heat to low. Mix in heavy cream and anchovy filets.

2.Bring the mixture back to medium heat, stirring from time to time, until bubbling. Serve hot.

Nutrition: Calories 670, Fat 34, Carbs 26, Protein 28, Sodium 430

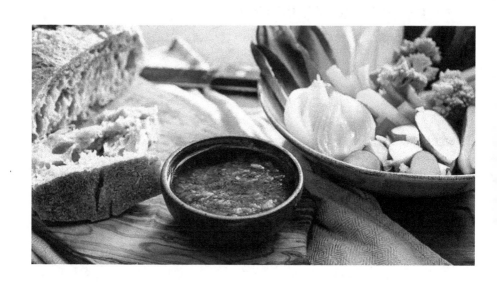

Bermuda Fish Chowder

Prep time: 10 min

Cook Time: 30 min

Serving: 2

Ingredients:

- 2 tablespoons vegetable oil
- 3 stalks celery, chopped
- 2 carrots, chopped
- 1 onion, chopped
- 1 green bell pepper, chopped
- 3 cloves garlic, minced
- 3 tablespoons tomato paste
- 4 cups clam juice
- 2 potatoes, peeled and cubed
- 1 (14.5 ounces) can peeled tomatoes
- 2 spoons Worcestershire sauce
- 1 jalapeno pepper
- 1 little spoon ground black pepper
- 1 bay-leaf
- 1 pound red-snapper fillets, cut into 1 inch pieces

Instructions:

1.In a large soup pot, heat the oil over medium heat. Toss in the carrots, celery, green pepper, onion, and garlic and sauté them for about 8 minutes.

2.Pour in the tomato paste and cook and stir for 1 minute. Mix in the clam juice, canned tomatoes with juice, potatoes, Worcestershire sauce, bay leaf, jalapeno pepper, and ground black pepper. Let it simmer until the potatoes are already tender, stirring the soup for about every 30 minutes.

3.Put the fish in and let it simmer for about 10 minutes until the snapper easily flakes with a fork.

Nutrition: Calories 320, Fat 28, Carbs 21, Protein 36, Sodium 660

Salmon Tikka

Prep time: 10 min

Cook Time: 30 min

Serving: 2

Ingredients:

- red pepper
- turmeric
- salt
- salmon fillets
- cornstarch
- oil

Instructions:

1.In a bowl, combine salt, turmeric, and cayenne. Put salmon into the bowl; toss until evenly coated with seasoning mixture. Let fish rest for 15 minutes.

2.In a container, heat oil over medium heat. Meanwhile, sprinkle cornstarch all over salmon; toss to coat evenly.

3.Cook salmon in hot oil, about 1 minute on each side, until golden brown.

Nutrition: Calories 254, Fat 24, Carbs 12, Protein 26, Sodium 765

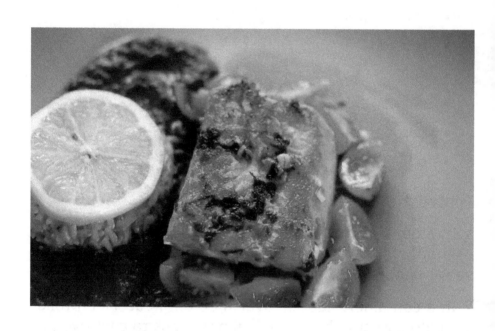

Almond And Parmesan Crusted Tilapia

Prep time: 10 min

Cook Time: 30 min

Serving: 2

Ingredients:

- 1 teaspoon olive oil, or as needed
- 3 cloves garlic, minced
- 1/2 cup grated Parmesan cheese
- almonds, crushed
- mayonnaise
- bread crumbs
- 2 tablespoons fresh lemon juice
- 1/4 teaspoon dried basil
- 1/4 teaspoon ground black pepper
- 1/8 teaspoon onion powder
- 1/8 teaspoon celery salt
- 1 pound tilapia fillets

Instructions:

1.Put the rack 6 inches away from the heat source and start preheating the oven's broiler. Use aluminum foil to line a broiling tray or use olive oil cooking spray to coat.

2.Heat olive oil in a frying container over medium heat, stir garlic while cooking for 3 to 5 minutes, or aromatic.

3.In a bowl, combine celery salt, onion powder, black pepper, basil, seafood seasoning, lemon juice, bread crumbs, mayonnaise, almonds, buttery spreads, garlic, and Parmesan cheese.

4.Set the tilapia fillets in a layer on top of the prepared pan, use aluminum foil to cover it.

5.Put the container in the preheated oven and start boiling for about 2 to 3 minutes. Flip the fillets, cover the pan with aluminum foil, and restart broiling for 2 to 3 more minutes. Remove aluminum foil and put the Parmesan cheese mixture on top to cover the fish. Broil in the oven for 2 more minutes until topping gets browned; fish can be shredded easily with a fork.

Nutrition: Calories 498, Fat 32, Carbs 26, Protein 8, Sodium 634

Crab And Shrimp Pasta Salad

Prep time: 10 min

Cook Time: 30 min

Serving: 2

Ingredients:

- 1 (16 ounces) package uncooked tri-colored spiral pasta
- 1/2 cup mayonnaise
- 1/4 cup apple cider vinegar
- 1/4 cup olive oil
- salt and pepper to taste
- 1 (8 ounces) package imitation crabmeat, flaked
- 1 (6.5 ounces) can tiny shrimp, drained
- 1-pint grape tomatoes halved
- 1 English cucumber, diced
- 1 (4 ounces) can slice black olives, drained
- 1 red bell pepper, seeded and chopped

Instructions:

1.Boil a big pot with lightly salted water. Add pasta. Cook for 10 minutes till tender, then drain. Cool by rinsing under cold water. Put into a big bowl, put aside.

2.Mix pepper, salt, olive oil, vinegar, and mayonnaise in a small bowl. Put on pasta; mix to coat. Add bell pepper, black olives, cucumber, tomatoes, shrimp, and crab. Gently mix to coat in dressing. Taste, then adjust seasoning if you want. Mix extra mayonnaise if the pasta is very dry.

Nutrition: Calories 480, Fat 24, Carbs 10, Protein 23, Sodium 680

Cream Of Salmon Soup

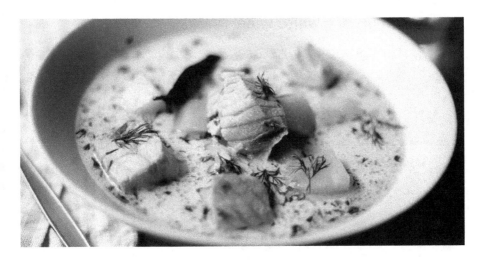

Prep time: 10 min

Cook Time: 30 min

Serving: 2

Ingredients:

Puff Pastry Triangles:

- 1 sheet frozen puff pastry, thawed
- 1 egg yolk, beaten
- 1 tablespoon sesame seeds

Salmon Soup:

- 1 1/2 tablespoons butter
- 1 onion, diced

- 18 ounces salmon fillets, diced
- 1 tablespoon tomato paste
- 2 1/2 cups fish stock
- 1/2 cup dry white wine
- 1 tablespoon cornstarch
- 1 1/4 cups heavy whipping cream
- A little saffron, salt and white pepper, freshly ground, to taste
- 3 little spoons chopped fresh dill

Instructions:

1.Set the oven at 400°F and start preheating.

2.On a lightly floured surface, place puff pastry; use a rolling pin to roll it out. Brush egg yolk over. Put sesame seeds on top; press in firmly. First, divide puff pastry into squares, then into triangles, put them on a baking sheet.

3.Start baking for about 15 minutes in the preheated oven till triangles are puffed up and golden brown.

4.In the meantime, place a pot on medium heat, melt in the butter and cook in onion till soft and translucent, about 5 minutes. 5.Include in salmon and cook for 5 minutes. Mix in tomato paste; cook for 1 minute. Add in white wine and fish stock. Boil everything; turn down the heat; simmer for 15 minutes. Let it boil.

6.Blend a little bit of water and cornstarch into a paste. Pour into the soup and let the mixture come to a boil. Cook till the soup is thickened, about 5 minutes. Make the soup into a smooth purée with an immersion blender. Mix in saffron and cream. Flavor with pepper and salt.

7.Dill for garnish and puff pastry triangles to serve with the soup.

Nutrition: Calories 436, Fat 32, Carbs 26, Protein 36, Sodium 663

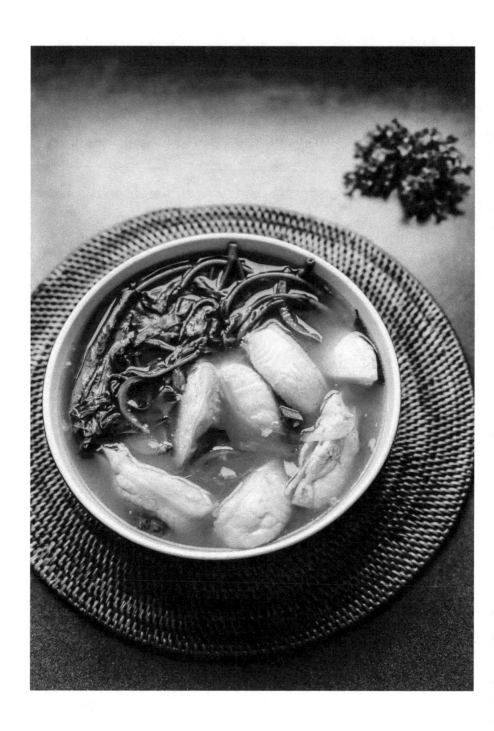

Creamed Salmon On Toast

Prep time: 10 min

Cook Time: 30 min

Serving: 2

Ingredients:

- Butter
- flour
- milk
- green peas
- 1 (14.75 ounces) can salmon
- salt and pepper to taste

Instructions:

1.Set the heat to medium, then melt butter in a skillet or saucepan. Whisk the flour while stirring continuously to have a smooth paste. Carefully pour the milk while stirring continuously with the peas' leftover liquids to make a smooth thick gravy.

2.Break large pieces of the salmon into smaller pieces by flaking them into a bowl. Mix the peas and salmon carefully into the sauce using a wooden spoon to keep the peas from being mashed. Cook until thoroughly heated.

3.Use a toaster oven or a broiler pan to toast some bread. You can even add butter if you want and garnish it with some salmon mixture on top.

Nutrition: Calories 244, Fat 32, Carbs 26, Protein 6, Sodium 321

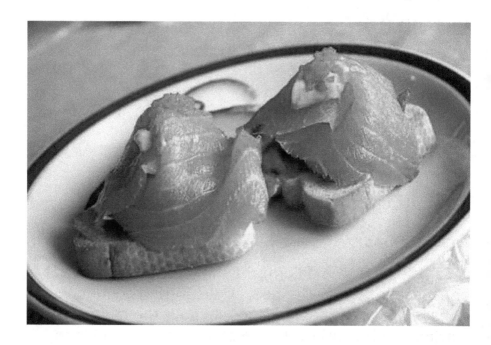

Coconut Salsa on Chipotle Fish Tacos

Prep Time: 10 minutes

Cook Time: 10 minutes

Serve: 4

Ingredients:

- ¼ cup chopped fresh cilantro
- ½ cup seeded and finely chopped plum tomato
- 1 cup peeled and finely chopped mango
- 1 lime cut into wedges
- 1 tablespoon chipotle Chile powder
- 1 tablespoon safflower oil
- 1/3 cup finely chopped red onion
- 10 tablespoon fresh lime juice, divided
- 4 6-oz boneless, skinless cod fillets
- 5 tablespoon dried unsweetened shredded coconut
- 8 pcs of 6-inch tortillas, heated

Instructions:

1. Whisk well Chile powder, oil, and 4 tablespoon lime juice in a glass baking dish. Add cod and marinate for 12 – 15 minutes. Turning once halfway through the marinating time.

2. Make the salsa by mixing coconut, 6 tablespoon lime juice, cilantro, onions, tomatoes and mangoes in a medium bowl. Set aside.

3. On high, heat a grill pan. Place cod and grill for four minutes per side, turning only once.

4. Once cooked, slice cod into large flakes and evenly divide onto the tortilla.

5. Evenly divide salsa on top of cod and serve with a side of lime wedges.

Nutrition: Calories: 477 Protein: 35.0g Fat: 12.4g Carbs: 57.4g

Baked Cod Crusted with Herbs

Prep Time: 5 minutes

Cook Time: 10 minutes

Serve: 4

Ingredients:

- ¼ cup honey
- ¼ teaspoon salt
- ½ cup panko
- ½ teaspoon pepper
- 1 tablespoon extra virgin olive oil
- 1 tablespoon lemon juice
- 1 teaspoon dried basil
- 1 teaspoon dried parsley
- 1 teaspoon rosemary
- 4 pieces of 4-oz cod fillets

Instructions:

1. With olive oil, grease a 9 x 13-inch baking pan and preheat oven to 375oF.

2. In a zip-top bag, mix panko, rosemary, salt, pepper, parsley and basil.

3. Evenly spread cod fillets in a prepped dish and drizzle with lemon juice.

4. Then brush the fillets with honey on all sides. Discard remaining honey, if any.

5. Then evenly divide the panko mixture on top of cod fillets.

6. Pop in the oven and bake for ten minutes or until fish is cooked.

Nutrition: Calories: 137 Protein: 5g Fat: 2g Carbs: 21g

Cajun Garlic Shrimp Noodle Bowl

Prep Time: 10 minutes

Cook Time: 15 minutes

Serve: 2

Ingredients:

- ½ teaspoon salt
- 1 onion, sliced
- 1 red pepper, sliced
- 1 tablespoon butter
- 1 teaspoon garlic granules
- 1 teaspoon onion powder
- 1 teaspoon paprika
- 2 large zucchinis, cut into noodle strips
- 20 jumbo shrimps, shells removed and deveined
- 3 cloves garlic, minced
- 3 tablespoon ghee
- A dash of cayenne pepper
- A dash of red pepper flakes

Instructions:

1. Prepare the Cajun seasoning by mixing the onion powder, garlic granules, pepper flakes, cayenne pepper, paprika and salt. Toss in the shrimp to coat in the seasoning.

2. In a skillet, heat the ghee and sauté the garlic. Add in the red pepper and onions and continue sautéing for 4 minutes.

3. Add the Cajun shrimp and cook until opaque. Set aside.

4. In another pan, heat the butter and sauté the zucchini noodles for three minutes.

5. Assemble by placing the Cajun shrimps on top of the zucchini noodles.

Nutrition: Calories: 712 Fat: 30.0g Protein: 97.8g Carbs: 20.2g

Crazy Saganaki Shrimp

Prep Time: 10 minutes

Cook Time: 10 minutes

Serve: 4

Ingredients:

- ¼ teaspoon salt
- ½ cup Chardonnay
- ½ cup crumbled Greek feta cheese
- 1 medium bulb. fennel, cored and finely chopped
- 1 small Chile pepper, seeded and minced
- 1 tablespoon extra virgin olive oil
- 12 jumbo shrimps, deveined with tails left on
- 2 tablespoon lemon juice, divided
- 5 scallions sliced thinly
- Pepper to taste

Instructions:

1. In a medium bowl, mix salt, lemon juice and shrimp.

2. On medium fire, place a saganaki pan (or large nonstick saucepan) and heat oil.

3. Sauté Chile pepper, scallions, and fennel for 4 minutes or until starting to brown and is already soft.

4. Add wine and sauté for another minute.

5. Place shrimps on top of the fennel, cover and cook for 4 minutes or until shrimps are pink.

6. Remove just the shrimp and transfer to a plate.

7. Add pepper, feta and 1 tablespoon lemon juice to the pan and cook for a minute or until cheese begins to melt.

8. To serve, place cheese and fennel mixture on a serving plate and top with shrimps.

Nutrition: Calories: 310 Protein: 49.7g Fat: 6.8g Carbs: 8.4g

Creamy Bacon-Fish Chowder

Prep Time: 10 minutes

Cook Time: 30 minutes

Serve: 8

Ingredients:

- 1 1/2 lbs. cod
- 1 1/2 teaspoon dried thyme
- 1 large onion, chopped
- 1 medium carrot, coarsely chopped
- 1 tablespoon butter, cut into small pieces
- 1 teaspoon salt, divided
- 3 1/2 cups baking potato, peeled and cubed
- 3 slices uncooked bacon
- 3/4 teaspoon ground black pepper, divided
- 4 1/2 cups water
- 4 bay leaves
- 4 cups 2% reduced-fat milk

Instructions:

1. In a large skillet, add the water and bay leaves and let it simmer. Add the fish. Cover and let it simmer some more until the flesh flakes easily with a fork. Remove the fish from the skillet and cut it into large pieces. Set aside the cooking liquid.

2. Place Dutch oven in medium heat and cook the bacon until crisp. Remove the bacon and reserve the bacon drippings. Crush the bacon and set aside.

3. Stir potato, onion and carrot in the pan with the bacon drippings, cook over medium heat for 10 minutes. Add the cooking liquid, bay leaves, 1/2 teaspoon salt, 1/4 teaspoon pepper and thyme, let it boil. Lower the heat and let simmer for 11 minutes. Add the milk and butter, simmer until the potatoes become tender, but do not boil. Add the fish, 1/2 teaspoon salt, 1/2 teaspoon pepper. Remove the bay leaves.

4. Serve sprinkled with the crushed bacon.

Nutrition: Calories: 400 Carbs: 34.5g Protein: 20.8g Fat: 19.7g

Crisped Coco-Shrimp with Mango Dip

Prep Time: 10 minutes

Cook Time: 20 minutes

Serve: 4

Ingredients:

- 1 cup shredded coconut
- 1 lb. raw shrimp, peeled and deveined
- 2 egg whites
- 4 tablespoon tapioca starch
- Pepper and salt to tast
- Mango Dip Ingredients:
- 1 cup mango, chopped
- 1 jalapeño, thinly minced
- 1 teaspoon lime juice
- 1/3 cup coconut milk
- 3 teaspoon raw honey

Instructions:

1. preheat oven to 400oF.

2. Ready a pan with a wire rack on top.

3. In a medium bowl, add tapioca starch and season with pepper and salt.

4. In a second medium bowl, add egg whites and whisk.

5. In a third medium bowl, add coconut.

6. To ready shrimps, dip first in tapioca starch, then egg whites, and then coconut. Place dredged shrimp on wire rack. Repeat until all shrimps are covered.

7. Pop shrimps in the oven and roast for 10 minutes per side.

8. Meanwhile, make the dip by adding all ingredients in a blender. Puree until smooth and creamy. Transfer to a dipping bowl.

9. Once shrimps are golden brown, serve with mango dip.

Nutrition: Calories: 294.2 Protein: 26.6g Fat: 7g Carbs: 31.2g

Cucumber-Basil Salsa on Halibut Pouches

Prep Time: 10 minutes

Cook Time: 17 minutes

Serve: 4

Ingredients:

- 1 lime, thinly sliced into eight pieces
- 2 cups mustard greens, stems removed
- 2 teaspoon olive oil
- 4 – 5 radishes trimmed and quartered
- 4 4-oz skinless halibut filets
- 4 large fresh basil leaves
- Cayenne pepper to taste – optional
- Pepper and salt to taste
- Salsa Ingredients:
- 1 ½ cups diced cucumber
- 1 ½ finely chopped fresh basil leaves
- 2 teaspoon fresh lime juice
- Pepper and salt to taste

Instructions:

1. preheat oven to 400°F.

2. Prepare parchment papers by making 4 pieces of 15 x 12-inch rectangles. Lengthwise, fold in half and unfold pieces on the table.

3. Season halibut fillets with pepper, salt and cayenne—if using cayenne.

4. Just to the right of the fold, place ½ cup of mustard greens. Add a basil leaf on the center of mustard greens and topped with 1 lime slice. Around the greens, layer ¼ of the radishes. Drizzle with ½ teaspoon of oil, season with pepper and salt. Top it with a slice of halibut fillet.

5. Just as you would make a calzone, fold the parchment paper over your filling and crimp the edges of the parchment paper beginning from one end to the other end. To seal the end of the crimped parchment paper, pinch it.

6. Repeat the remaining ingredients until you have 4 pieces of parchment papers filled with halibut and greens.

7. Place pouches in a pan and bake in the oven until halibut is flaky around 15 to 17 minutes.

8. While waiting for halibut pouches to cook, make your salsa by mixing all salsa ingredients in a medium bowl.

9. Once halibut is cooked, remove it from the oven and make a tear on top. Be careful of the steam as it is very hot. Equally, divide salsa and spoon ¼ of salsa on top of halibut through the slit you have created.

Nutrition: Calories: 335.4 Protein: 20.2g Fat: 16.3g
Carbs: 22.1g

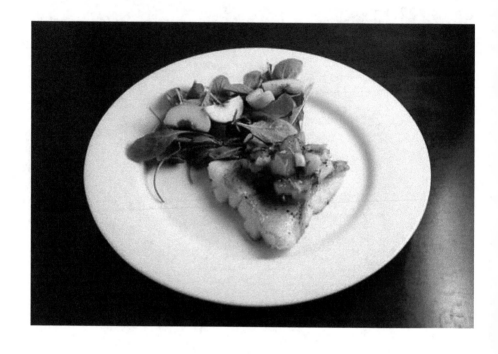

Salmon with Mustard

Prep Time: 10 minutes

Cook Time: 8 minutes

Serve: 4

Ingredients:

- ¼ teaspoon ground red pepper or chili powder
- ¼ teaspoon ground turmeric
- ¼ teaspoon salt
- 1 teaspoon honey
- 1/8 teaspoon garlic powder or a minced clove garlic

  2 teaspoon. whole grain mustard 4 pcs 6-oz salmon fillets

Instructions:

1. In a small bowl, mix well salt, garlic powder, red pepper, turmeric, honey and mustard.

2. Preheat the oven to broil and grease a baking dish with cooking spray.

3. Place salmon on a baking dish with skin side down and spread evenly mustard mixture on top of salmon.

4. Pop in the oven and broil until flaky, around 8 minutes.

Nutrition: Calories: 324 Fat: 18.9 g Protein: 34 g Carbs: 2.9g

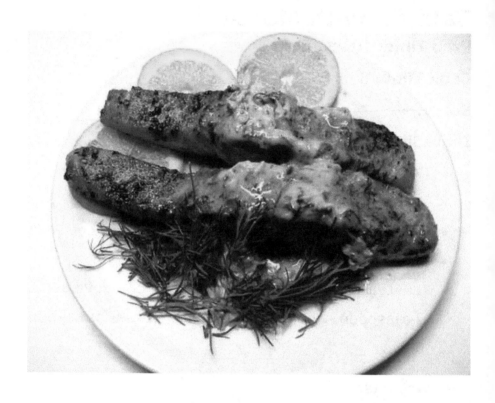

Dijon Mustard and Lime Marinated Shrimp

Prep Time: 10 minutes

Cook Time: 10 minutes

Serve: 8

Ingredients:

- ½ cup fresh lime juice and lime zest as garnish
- ½ cup of rice vinegar
- ½ teaspoon hot sauce
- 1 bay leaf
- 1 cup of water
- 1 lb. uncooked shrimp, peeled and deveined
- 1 medium red onion, chopped
- 2 tablespoon capers
- 2 tablespoon Dijon mustard
- 3 whole cloves

Instructions:

1. Mix hot sauce, mustard, capers, lime juice and onion in a shallow baking dish and set aside.

2. Put the bay leaf, cloves, vinegar, and water to a boil in a large saucepan.

3. Once boiling, add shrimps and cook for a minute while stirring continuously.

4. Drain shrimps and pour shrimps into onion mixture.

5. For an hour, refrigerate while covered the shrimps.

6. Then serve shrimps cold and garnished with lime zest.

Nutrition: Calories: 232.2 Protein: 17.8g Fat: 3g Carbs: 15g

Dill Relish on White Sea Bass

Prep Time: 10 minutes

Cook Time: 12 minutes

Serve: 4

Ingredients:

- 1 ½ tablespoon chopped white onion
- 1 ½ teaspoon chopped fresh dill
- 1 lemon, quartered
- 1 teaspoon Dijon mustard
- 1 teaspoon lemon juice
- 1 teaspoon pickled baby capers, drained
- 4 pieces of 4-oz white sea bass fillets

Instructions:

1. Preheat oven to 375°F.

2. Mix lemon juice, mustard, dill, capers and onions in a small bowl.

3. Prepare four aluminum foil squares and place 1 fillet per foil.

4. Squeeze a lemon wedge per fish.

5. Evenly divide into 4 the dill spread and drizzle over the fillet.

6. Close the foil over the fish securely and pop in the oven.

7. Bake for 12 minutes or until fish is cooked through.

8. Remove from foil and transfer to a serving platter.

Nutrition: Calories: 115 Protein: 7g Fat: 1g Carbs: 12g

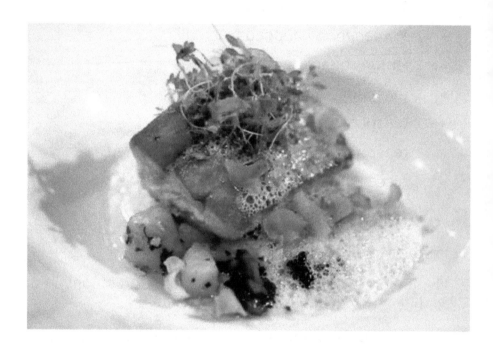

Salmon & Arugula Omelet

Prep Time: 10 minutes

Cook Time: 7 minutes

Serve: 4

Ingredients:

- 6 eggs
- 2 tablespoons unsweetened almond milk Salt and ground black pepper, as required 2 tablespoons olive oil
- 4 ounces smoked salmon, cut into bite-sized chunks
- 2 cups fresh arugula, chopped finely
- 4 scallions, chopped finely

Instructions:

1.In a bowl, place the eggs, coconut milk, salt and black pepper and beat well. Set aside.

2. Over medium pressure, heat the oil in a non-stick skillet.

3.Place the egg mixture evenly and cook for about 30 seconds without stirring.

4.Place the salmon kale and scallions on top of egg mixture evenly.

5. Lower the heat to a low level and cook covered for about 4-5 minutes or until omelet is done completely.

6.Uncover the skillet and cook for about 1 minute.

7.Carefully transfer the omelet onto a serving plate.

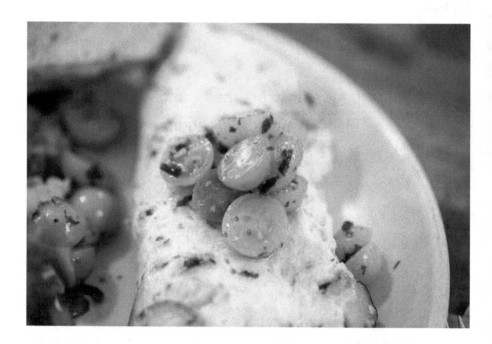

Tuna Omelet

Prep Time: 10 minutes

Cook Time: 5 minutes

Serve: 2

Ingredients:

- 4 eggs
- ¼ cup unsweetened almond milk
- 1 tablespoon scallions, chopped
- 1 garlic clove, minced
- ½ of jalapeño pepper, minced
- Salt and ground black pepper, to taste
- 1 (5-ounce) can water-packed tuna, drained and flaked
- 1 tablespoon olive oil
- 3 normal spoons green bell pepper, seeded and chopped
- 3 tablespoons tomato, chopped
- ¼ cup low-fat cheddar cheese, shredded

Instructions:

1. In a bowl, add the eggs, almond milk, scallions, garlic, jalapeño pepper, salt, and black pepper, and beat well.

2. Add the tuna and stir to combine.

3.In a big-non-stick frying pan, heat oil over medium heat.

4.Place the egg mixture in an even layer and cook for about 1–2 minutes, without stirring.

5.Carefully lift the edges to run the uncooked portion flow underneath.

6.Spread the veggies over the egg mixture and sprinkle with the cheese.

7.Cover the frying pan and cook for about 30–60 seconds.

8.Remove the lid and fold the omelet in half.

9.Remove from the heat and cut the omelet into 2 portions.

Fish Stew

Prep Time: 15 minutes

Cook Time: 50 minutes

Serve: 10

Ingredients:

- ¼ cup coconut oil
- ½ cup yellow onion, chopped
- 1 cup celery stalk, chopped
- ½ cup green bell pepper, seeded and chopped
- 1 garlic clove, minced
- 4 cups water
- 4 beef bouillon cubes
- 20 ounces okra, trimmed and chopped
- 2 (14-ounce) cans sugar-free diced tomatoes with liquid
- 2 bay leaves
- 1 teaspoon dried thyme, crushed
- 2 teaspoons red pepper flakes, crushed
- ¼ teaspoon hot pepper sauce
- Salt and ground black pepper, as required
- 32 ounces catfish fillets
- ½ cup fresh cilantro, chopped

Instructions:

1.In a big skillet, melt the coconut oil over medium heat and sauté the onion, celery and bell pepper for about 4-5 minutes.

2.Meanwhile, in a large soup pan, mix together bouillon cubes and water and bring to a boil over medium heat.

3.Transfer the onion mixture and remaining ingredients except catfish into the pan of boiling water and bring to a boil.

4.Decrease the heat to low, cook for about 30 minutes, protected.

5.Stir in catfish fillets and cook for about 10-15 minutes.

6. Stir in the cilantro and remove from the heat.

Salmon & Veggie Salad

Prep Time: 15 minutes

Serve: 2

Ingredients:

- 6 ounces cooked wild salmon, chopped
- 1 cup cucumber, sliced
- 1 cup red bell-pepper, seeded and sliced ½ cup grape tomatoes, quartered
- 1 tablespoon scallion green, chopped
- 1 cup lettuce, torn
- 1 cup fresh spinach, torn
- 2 tablespoons olive oil
- 2 tablespoons fresh lemon juice

Instructions:

1.In a salad bowl, place all ingredients and gently toss to coat well.

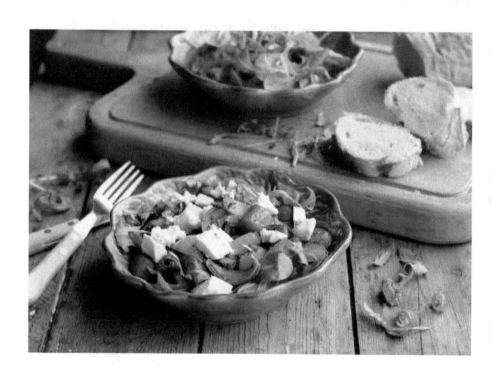

Tuna Salad

Prep Time: 15 minutes

Serve: 4

Ingredients:

For Dressing:

- 2 tablespoons fresh dill, minced
- 2 tablespoons olive oil
- 1 tablespoon fresh lime juice
- Salt and ground black pepper, to taste

For Salad:

- 4 cups fresh spinach, torn
- 2 (6-ounce) cans water-packed tuna, drained and flaked
- 6 hard-boiled eggs, peeled and sliced
- 1 cup tomato, chopped
- 1 large cucumber, sliced

Instructions:

1. For Dressing: place dill, oil, lime juice, salt, and black pepper in a small bowl and beat until well combined.

2. Divide the spinach onto serving plates and top each with tuna, egg, cucumber, and tomato.

3. Drizzle with dressing.

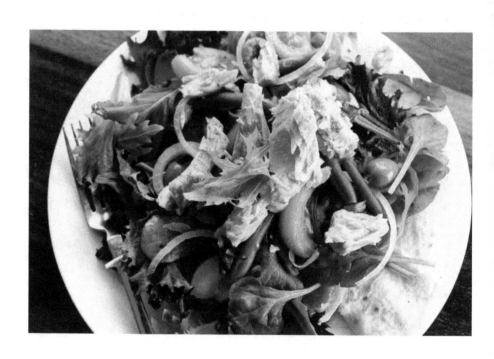

Shrimp & Greens Salad

Prep Time: 15 minutes

Cook Time: 6 minutes

Serve: 6

Ingredients:

- 3 tablespoons olive oil, divided
- 1 garlic clove, crushed and divided
- 2 tablespoons fresh rosemary, chopped
- 1-pound shrimp, peeled and deveined
- Salt and ground black pepper, as required
- 4 cups fresh arugula
- 2 cups lettuce, torn
- 2 tablespoons fresh lime juice

Instructions:

1.In a large wok, heat 1 normal spoon of oil over medium heat and sauté 1 garlic clove for about 1 minute.

2.Add the shrimp with salt and black pepper and cook for about 4-5 minutes.

3. Remove from the heat and place to cool aside.

4.Ina large bowl, add the shrimp, arugula, remaining oil, lime juice, salt and black pepper and gently, toss to coat.

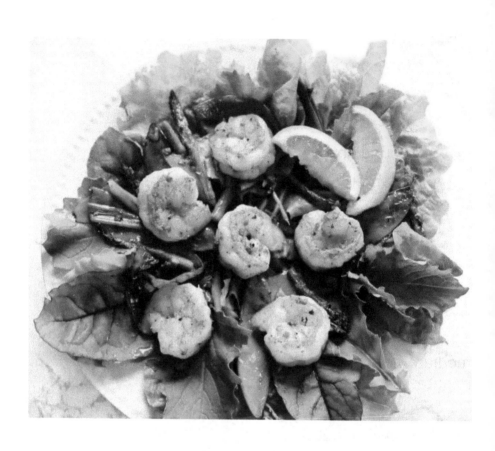

Shrimp, Apple & Carrot Salad

Prep Time: 20 minutes

Cook Time: 3 minutes

Serve: 4

Ingredients:

- 12 medium shrimp
- 1½ cups Granny Smith apple, cored and sliced thinly 1½ cups carrot, peeled and cut into matchsticks
- ½ cup fresh mint leaves, chopped
- 2 tablespoons balsamic vinegar
- ¼ cup extra-virgin olive oil
- 1 teaspoon lemongrass, chopped
- 1 teaspoon garlic, minced
- 2 sprigs fresh cilantro, leaves separated and chopped

Instructions:

1.In a large pan of the salted boiling water, add the shrimp and lemon and cook for about 3 minutes.

2.Remove from the heat and drain the shrimp well.

3.Set aside to cool.

4.After cooling, peel and devein the shrimps.

5.Transfer the shrimp into a large bowl.

6.Add the remaining all ingredients except cilantro and gently, stir to combine.

7.Cover the bowl and refrigerate for about 1 hour.

8.Top with cilantro just before serving.

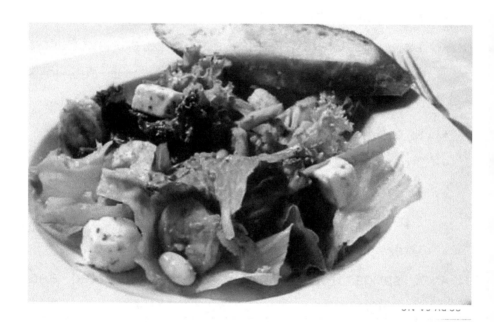

Shrimp & Green Beans Salad

Prep Time: 20 minutes

Cook Time: 8 minutes

Serve: 5

Ingredients:

For Shrimp:

- 2 tablespoons olive oil
- 2 tablespoons fresh key lime juice
- 4 large garlic cloves, peeled
- 2 sprigs fresh rosemary leaves
- ½ teaspoon garlic salt
- 20 large shrimp, peeled and deveined

For Salad:

- 1-pound fresh green beans, trimmed
- ¼ cup olive oil
- 1 onion, sliced
- Salt and ground black pepper, as required ½ cup garlic and herb feta cheese, crumbled

Instructions:

1.For shrimp marinade: in a blender, add all the ingredients except shrimp and pulse until smooth.

2.Transfer the marinade in a large bowl.

3.Add the shrimp and coat with marinade generously.

4. Cover the bowl and refrigerate for a minimum of 31 minutes to marinate.

5.Preheat the broiler of oven. Arrange the rack in top position of the oven. Line a large baking sheet with a piece of foil.

6.Place the shrimp with marinade onto the prepared baking sheet.

7.Broil for about 3-4 minutes per side.

8.Transfer the shrimp mixture into a bowl and refrigerate until using.

9.Meanwhile, For Salad: in a pan of the salted boiling water, add the green beans and cook for about 3-4 minutes.

10.Drain the green beans well and rinse under cold running water.

11.Transfer the green beans into a large bowl.

12.Add the onion, shrimp, salt and black pepper and stir to combine.

13.Cover and refrigerate to chill for about 1 hour.

14.Stir in cheese just before serving.

Shrimp & Olives Salad

Prep Time: 15 minutes

Cook Time: 3 minutes

Serve: 4

Ingredients:

- 1-pound shrimp, peeled and deveined
- 1 lemon, quartered
- 2 tablespoons olive oil
- 2 teaspoons fresh lemon juice
- Salt and freshly ground-black-pepper, to taste
- 2 tomatoe, sliced
- ¼ cup onion, sliced
- ¼ cup green olives
- ¼ cup fresh cilantro, chopped finely

Instructions:

1. In a tub of boiling water that is finely salted, add the quartered lemon.

2. Then, add the shrimp and cook for about 2-3 minutes or until pink and opaque.

3. With a slotted spoon, transfer the shrimp into a bowl of ice water to stop the cooking process.

4. Drain the shrimp completely and then pat dry with paper towels.

5.In a small bowl, add the oil, lemon juice, salt, and black pepper, and beat until well combined.

6.Divide the shrimp, tomato, onion, olives, and cilantro onto serving plates.

7.Drizzle with oil mixture.

Shrimp & Arugula Salad

Prep Time: 15 minutes

Cook Time: 5 minutes

Serve: 4

Ingredients:

For Shrimp:

- 1-pound large shrimp, peeled and deveined ½ tablespoon fresh lemon juice

For Salad:

- 6 cups fresh arugula
- 2 tablespoons extra-virgin olive oil
- 1 tablespoons fresh lemon juice
- Salt and ground black pepper, as required

Instructions:

1.In a large pan of salted boiling water, add the shrimp and lemon juice and cook for about 2 minutes.

2. Withdraw the shrimp from the pan with a slotted-spoon and put it in an ice bath.

3.Drain the shrimp well.

4.In a large bowl, add the shrimp, arugula, oil, lemon juice, salt and black pepper and gently, toss to coat.

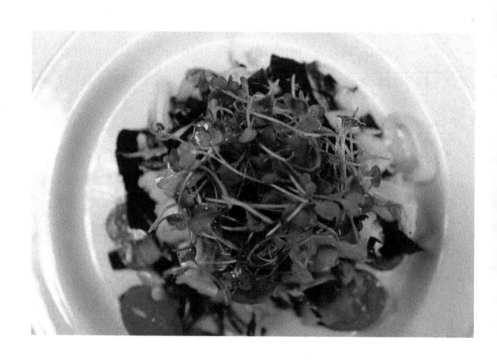

Shrimp & Veggies Salad

Prep Time: 20 minutes

Cook Time: 5 minutes

Serve: 6

Ingredients:

For Dressing:

- 2 tablespoons natural almond butter
- 1 garlic clove, crushed
- 1 tablespoon fresh cilantro, chopped
- 2 tablespoons fresh lime juice
- 1 tablespoon maple syrup
- ½ teaspoon cayenne pepper
- ¼ teaspoon salt
- 1 tablespoon water
- 1/3 cup olive oil

For Salad:

- 1-pound shrimp, peeled and deveined Salt and ground black pepper, as required
- 1 teaspoon olive oil
- 1 cup carrot, peeled and julienned
- 1 cup red cabbage, shredded
- 1 cup green cabbage, shredded
- 1 cup cucumber, julienned

- 4 cups fresh baby arugula
- ¼ cup fresh basil, chopped
- ¼ cup fresh cilantro, chopped
- 4 cups lettuce, torn
- ¼ cup almonds, chopped

Instructions:

1.For Dressing: in a bowl, add all ingredients except oil and beat until well combined.

2.Slowly, add oil, beating continuously until smooth.

3.For Salad: in a bowl, add shrimp, salt, black pepper and oil and toss to coat well.

4. Heat a skillet over medium-high heat and cook the shrimp on each side for about two minutes.

5.Detach from the heat to cool and set aside.

6.In a large serving bowl, add all the cooked shrimp, remaining salad ingredients and dressing and toss to coat well.

Salmon Lettuce Wraps

Prep Time: 10 minutes

Serve: 2

Ingredients:

- ¼ cup low-fat mozzarella cheese, cubed ¼ cup tomato, chopped
- 2 tablespoons fresh dill, chopped
- 1 teaspoon fresh lemon juice
- Salt, as required
- 4 lettuce leaves
- 1/3 pound cooked salmon, chopped

Instructions:

1.In a small bowl, combine mozzarella, tomato, dill, lemon juice, and salt until well combined.

2.Arrange the lettuce leaves onto serving plates.

3.Divide the salmon and tomato mixture over each lettuce leaf and serve immediately.

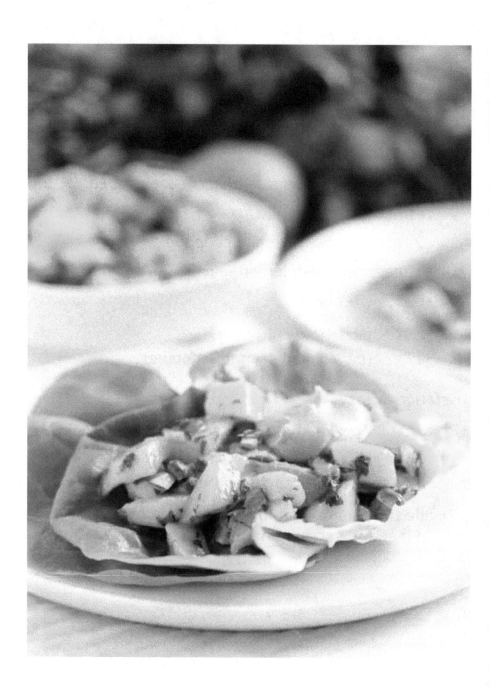

Tuna Burgers

Prep Time: 15 minutes

Cook Time: 6 minutes

Serve: 2

Ingredients:

- 1 (15-ounce) can water-packed tuna, drained
- ½ celery stalk, chopped
- 2 tablespoon fresh parsley, chopped
- 1 teaspoon fresh dill, chopped
- 2 tablespoon walnuts, chopped
- 2 tablespoon mayonnaise
- 1 egg, beaten
- 1 tablespoon butter
- 3 cups lettuce

Instructions:

1.For Burgers: add all ingredients except the butter and lettuce in a bowl and mix until well combined.

2.Make 2 equal-sized patties from mixture.

3.In a frying pan, melt butter over medium heat and cook the patties for about 2-3 minutes.

4.Carefully flip the side and cook for about 2-3 minutes.

5.Divide the lettuce onto serving plates.

6.Top each plate with 1 burger and serve.

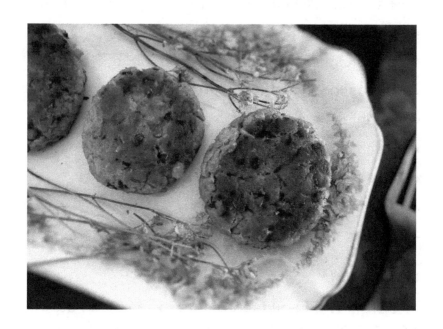

Spicy Salmon

Prep Time: 105 minutes

Cook Time: 8 minutes

Serve: 4

Ingredients:

- 4 tablespoons extra-virgin olive oil, divided
- 2 tablespoons fresh lemon juice
- 1 teaspoon ground turmeric
- 1 teaspoon ground cumin
- Salt and ground black pepper, as required
- 4 (4-ounce) boneless, skinless salmon fillets
- 6 cups fresh arugula

Instructions:

1.In a bowl, mix together 2 normal spoons of oil, lemon juice, turmeric, cumin, salt and black pepper.

2.Add the salmon fillets and coat with the oil mixture generously. Set aside.

3.In a non-stick wok, heat remaining oil over medium heat.

4.Place salmon fillets, skin-side down and cook for about 3-5 minutes.

5.Change the side and cook for about 2-3 minutes more.

6.Divide the salmon onto serving plates and serve immediately alongside the arugula.

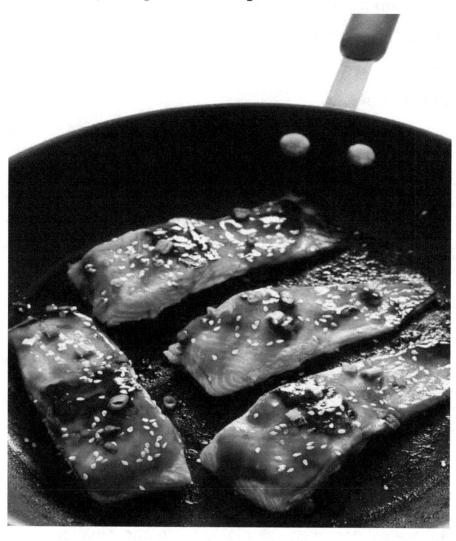

Lemony Salmon

Prep Time: 10 minutes

Cook Time: 14 minutes

Serve: 4

Ingredients:

- 2 garlic cloves, minced
- 1 tablespoon fresh lemon zest, grated
- 2 tablespoons olive oil
- 2 tablespoons fresh lemon juice
- Salt and ground black pepper, to taste
- 4 (6-ounce) boneless, skinless salmon fillets
- 6 cups fresh spinach

Instructions:

1. Preheat the grill to medium-high heat.

2.Grease the grill grate.

3.In a bowl, place all-ingredients except for salmon and spinach and mix well.

4.Add the salmon fillets and coat with garlic mixture generously.

5.Grill the salmon fillets for about 6-7 minutes per side.

6.Serve immediately alongside the spinach.

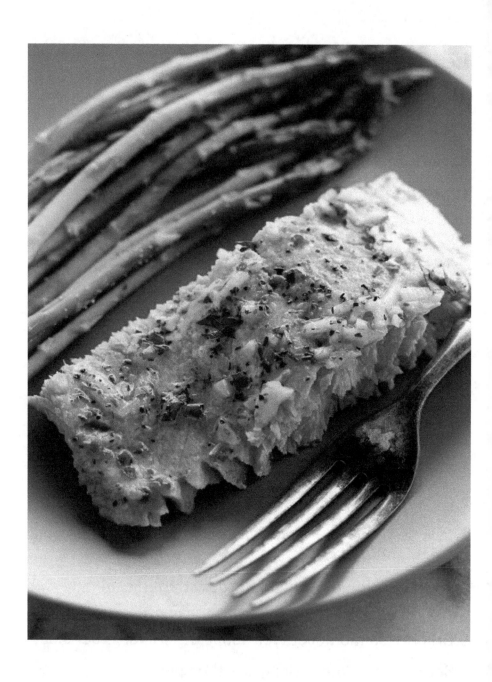

Zesty Salmon

Prep Time: 10 minutes

Cook Time: 10 minutes

Serve: 4

Ingredients:

- 1 tablespoon butter, melted
- 1 tablespoon fresh lemon juice
- 1 teaspoon Worcestershire sauce
- 1 teaspoon lemon zest, grated finely.
- 4 (6-ounce) salmon fillets
- Salt and ground black pepper, to taste

Instructions:

1.In a baking dish, place butter, lemon juice, Worcestershire sauce, and lemon zest, and mix well.

2.Coat the fillets with mixture and then arrange skin side-up in the baking dish.

3.Set aside for about 15 minutes.

4.Preheat the broiler of oven.

5.Arrange the oven rack about 6-inch from heating element.

6.Line a broiler pan with a piece of foil.

7.Remove the salmon fillets from baking dish and season with salt and black pepper.

8.Arrange the salmon fillets onto the prepared broiler pan, skin side down.

9.Broil for about 8-10 minutes.

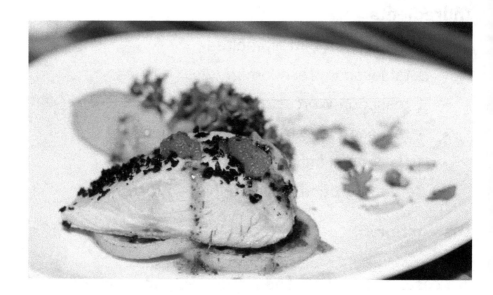

Stuffed Salmon

Prep Time: 15 minutes

Cook Time: 16 minutes

Serve: 4

Ingredients:

For Salmon:

- 4 (6-ounce) skinless salmon fillets
- Salt and ground black pepper, as required
- 2 tablespoons fresh lemon juice
- 2 tablespoons olive oil, divided
- 1 tablespoon unsalted butter

For Filling:

- 4 ounces low-fat cream cheese, softened
- ¼ cup low-fat Parmesan cheese, grated finely
- 4 ounces frozen spinach, thawed and squeezed
- 2 teaspoons garlic, minced
- Salt and ground black pepper, as required

Instructions:

1.Season each salmon-fillet with salt and black-pepper and then, drizzle with lemon juice and 1 tablespoon of oil.

2.Arrange the salmon fillets onto a smooth surface.

3.With a sharp knife, cut a pocket into each salmon fillet about ¾ of the way through, take care not to cut the whole way.

4.For filling: in a bowl, add the cream cheese, Parmesan cheese, spinach, garlic, salt and black pepper and mix well.

5.Place about 1-2 tablespoons of spinach mixture into each salmon pocket and spread evenly.

6.In a skillet, heat the remaining oil and butter over medium-high heat and cook the salmon fillets for about 6-8 minutes per side.

7.Remove the salmon fillets from heat and transfer onto the serving plates.

Salmon with Asparagus

Prep Time: 10 minutes

Cook Time: 20 minutes

Serve: 6

Ingredients:

- 6 (4-ounce) salmon fillets
- 2 tablespoons extra-virgin olive oil
- 3 tablespoons fresh parsley, minced
- ¼ teaspoon ginger powder
- Salt and freshly ground black-pepper, to taste
- 1½ pounds fresh asparagus

Instructions:

1. Preheat your oven to 400 degrees.

2. Grease a large baking dish.

3. In a bowl, place all-ingredients and mix well.

4. Arrange the salmon fillets into prepared baking dish in a single layer.

5. Bake for approximately 16-21 minutes or until desired doneness of salmon.

6. Meanwhile, in a pan of the boiling water, add asparagus and cook for about 4-5 minutes.

7. Drain the asparagus well.

8. Divide the asparagus onto serving plates evenly and top each with 1 salmon fillet and serve.

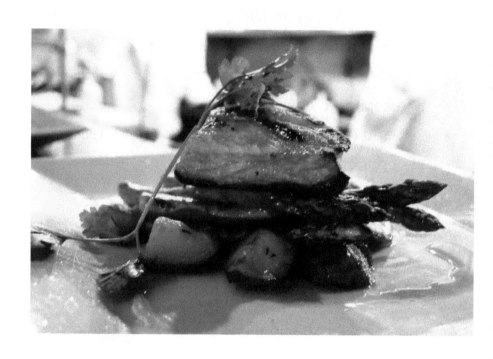

Salmon Parcel

Prep Time: 15 minutes

Cook Time: 20 minutes

Serve: 6

Ingredients:

- 6 (4-ounce) salmon-fillets
- Salt and freshly ground-black-pepper, to taste 1 yellow bell pepper, seeded and cubed
- 1 red bell pepper, seeded and cubed
- 4 plum tomatoes, cubed
- 1 small onion, sliced thinly
- ½ cup fresh parsley, chopped
- ¼ cup extra-virgin olive oil
- 2 tablespoons fresh lemon juice

Instructions:

1. Preheat your oven to 400 degrees F.

2. Arrange 6 pieces of foil onto a smooth surface.

3. Place one salmon-fillet on each piece of foil and sprinkle with salt and black pepper.

4. In a bowl, mix together bell peppers, tomato and onion.

5. Place veggie mixture over each fillet evenly and top with parsley and capers evenly.

6. Drizzle with oil and lemon juice.

7.Fold the each piece of foil around salmon mixture to seal it.

8.Arrange the foil packets onto a large baking sheet in a single layer.

9.Bake for approximately 25 minutes.

10.Remove from the oven and place the foil packets onto serving plates.

11.Carefully unwrap each foil packet and serve.

Salmon with Cauliflower Mash

Prep Time: 15 minutes

Cook Time: 20 minutes

Serve: 4

Ingredients:

For Cauliflower Mash:

- 1-pound cauliflower, cut into florets
- 1 tablespoon extra-virgin olive oil
- 3 garlic cloves, minced
- 1 teaspoon fresh thyme leaves
- Salt and freshly ground black-pepper, to taste

For Salmon:

- 1 (1-inch) piece fresh ginger, grated finely
- 1 tablespoon honey
- 1 tablespoon fresh lemon juice
- 1 tablespoon Dijon mustard
- 2 tablespoons olive oil
- 4 (6-ounce) salmon fillets
- 2 tablespoons fresh parsley, chopped

Instructions:

1.For mash: in a large saucepan of water, arrange a steamer basket and bring to a boil.

2.Place the cauliflower florets in steamer basket and steam covered for about 10 minutes.

3.Drain the cauliflower and set aside.

4.In a small-frying pan, heat the oil over-medium heat and sauté the garlic for about 2 minutes.

5.Remove the frying pan from heat and transfer the garlic oil in a large food processor.

6.Add the cauliflower, thyme, salt and black-pepper and pulse until smooth.

7.Transfer the cauliflower mash into a bowl and set aside.

8.Meanwhile, in a bowl, mix together ginger, honey, lemon juice and Dijon mustard. Set aside.

9.In a large non-stick skillet, heat olive-oil over medium-high heat and cook the salmon fillets for about 3-4 minutes per side.

10.Stir in honey mixture and immediately remove from heat.

11.Divide warm cauliflower mash onto serving plates.

12. Top each plate with one salmon fillet and serve.

Salmon with Salsa

Prep Time: 15 minutes

Cook Time: 8 minutes

Serve: 4

Ingredients:

For Salsa:

- 2 large ripe avocados, peeled, pitted and cut into small chunks
- 1 small tomato, chopped
- 2 tablespoons red onion, chopped finely ¼ cup fresh cilantro, chopped finely
- 1 tablespoon jalapeño pepper, seeded and minced finely
- 1 garlic clove, minced finely
- 3 tablespoon fresh lime juice
- Salt and ground black pepper, as required

For Salmon:

- 4 (5-ounce) (1-inch thick) salmon fillets
- Sea salt and ground black-pepper, as required
- 3 tablespoons olive oil
- 1 tablespoon fresh rosemary leaves, chopped
- 1 tablespoon fresh lemon juice

Instructions:

1.For salsa: add all ingredients in a bowl and gently, stir to combine.

2.With a plastic-wrap, cover the bowl and refrigerate before serving.

3.For salmon: season each salmon fillet with salt and black pepper generously.

4.In a big-skillet, heat the oil over medium-high heat.

5.Place the salmon fillets, skins side up and cook for about 4 minutes.

6.Carefully change the side of each salmon fillet and cook for about 4 minutes more.

7.Stir in the rosemary and lemon juice and remove from the heat.

8.Divide the salsa onto serving plates evenly.

9.To each plate with 1 salmon fillet and serve.

Walnut Crusted Salmon

Prep Time: 15 minutes

Cook Time: 20 minutes

Serve: 2

Ingredients:

- ½ cup walnuts
- 1 tablespoon fresh dill, chopped
- 2 tablespoons fresh lemon rind, grated
- Salt and ground black pepper, as required
- 1 tablespoon coconut oil, melted
- 3-4 tablespoons Dijon mustard
- 4 (3-ounce) salmon fillets
- 4 teaspoons fresh lemon juice
- 3 cups fresh baby spinach

Instructions:

1. Preheat your oven to 350 degrees F.

2. Line the parchment paper with a large baking sheet.

3. Place the walnuts in a food processor and pulse until chopped roughly.

4. Add the dill, lemon rind, garlic salt, black pepper, and butter, and pulse until a crumbly mixture forms.

5. Place the salmon fillets onto prepared baking sheet in a single layer, skin-side down.

6. Coat the top of each salmon-fillet with Dijon mustard.

7.Place the walnut mixture over each fillet and gently, press into the surface of salmon.

8.Bake for approximately 15–20 minutes.

9.Remove the salmon fillets from oven and transfer onto the serving plates.

10. Drizzle with the lemon juice and serve alongside the spinach.

Garlicky Tilapia

Prep Time: 10 minutes

Cook Time: 5 minutes

Serve: 4

Ingredients:

- 2 tablespoons olive oil
- 4 (5-ounce) tilapia fillets
- 3 garlic cloves, minced
- 1 tablespoon fresh ginger, minced
- 2-3 tablespoons low-sodium chicken broth Salt and ground black pepper, to taste
- 6 cups fresh baby spinach

Instructions:

1.In a big sauté-pan, heat the oil over medium heat and cook the tilapia fillets for about 3 minutes.

2.Flip the side and stir in the garlic and ginger.

3.Cook for about 1-2 minutes.

4.Add the broth and cook for about 2-3 more minutes.

5.Stir in salt and black pepper and remove from heat.

6.Serve hot alongside the spinach.

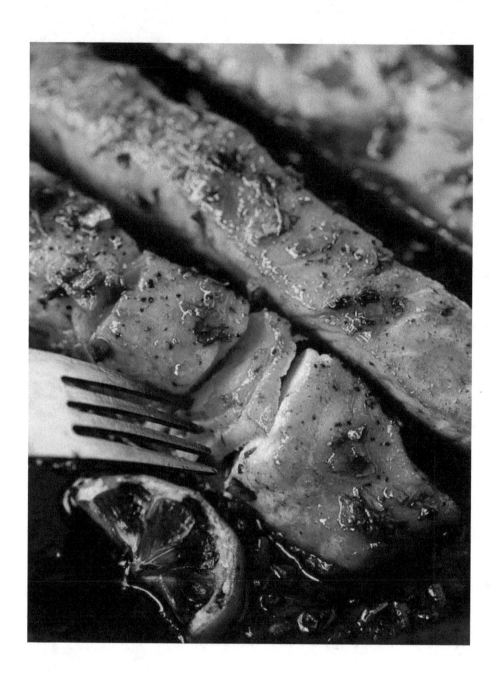

Tilapia Piccata

Prep Time: 15 minutes

Cook Time: 8 minutes

Serve: 4

Ingredients:

- 3 tablespoons fresh lemon juice
- 2 tablespoons olive oil
- 2 garlic cloves, minced
- ½ teaspoon lemon zest, grated
- 2 teaspoons capers, drained
- 2 tablespoons fresh basil, minced
- 4 (6-ounce) tilapia fillets
- Salt and ground black pepper, as required 6 cups fresh baby kale

Instructions:

1.Preheat the broiler of the oven.

2.Arrange an oven rack about 4-inch from the heating element.

3.Grease a broiler pan.

4.In a little-bowl, add the lemon juice, oil, garlic and lemon zest and beat until well combined.

5.Add the capers and basil and stir to combine.

6.Reserve 2 tablespoons of mixture in a small bowl.

7.Coat the fish fillets with remaining capers mixture and sprinkle with salt and black pepper.

8.Place the tilapia fillets onto the broiler pan and broil for about 3-4 minutes side.

9.Remove from the oven and place the fish fillets onto serving plates.

10. Drizzle with reserved capers mixture and serve alongside the kale.

Cod in Dill Sauce

Prep Time: 10 minutes

Cook Time: 13 minutes

Serve: 2

Ingredients:

- 2 (6-ounce) cod fillets
- 1 teaspoon onion powder
- Salt and ground black pepper, as required 3 tablespoons butter, divided
- 2 garlic cloves, minced
- 1-2 lemon slices
- 2 teaspoons fresh dill weed
- 3 cups fresh spinach, torn

Instructions:

1.Season each cod fillet evenly with the onion powder, salt and black pepper.

2.In a medium skillet, heat 1 normal spoon of oil over high heat and cook the cod fillets for about 4-5 minutes per side.

3.Transfer the cod fillets onto a plate.

4.Meanwhile, in a frying-pan, heat the remaining oil over low heat and sauté the garlic and lemon slices for about 40-60 seconds.

5.Stir in the cooked cod fillets and dill and cook, covered for about 1-2 minutes.

6.Remove the cod fillets from heat and transfer onto the serving plates.

7.Top with the pan sauce and serve immediately alongside the spinach.

Cod & Veggies Bake

Prep Time: 15 minutes

Cook Time: 20 minutes

Serve: 4

Ingredients:

- 1 teaspoon olive oil
- ½ cup onion, minced
- 1 cup zucchini, chopped
- 1 garlic clove, minced
- 2 tablespoons fresh basil, chopped
- 2 cups fresh tomatoes, chopped
- Salt and ground black pepper, as required
- 4 (6-ounce) cod steaks
- 1/3 cup feta cheese, crumbled

Instructions:

1. Preheat your oven to 450 degrees F.

2. Grease a large shallow baking dish.

3. In a skillet, heat oil over-medium heat and sauté the onion, zucchini and garlic for about 4-5 minutes.

4. Stir in the basil, tomatoes, salt and black pepper and immediately remove from heat.

5. Place the cod steaks into prepared baking dish in a single layer and top with tomato mixture evenly.

6. Sprinkle with the cheese evenly.

7.Bake for approximately 16 minutes or until desired doneness.

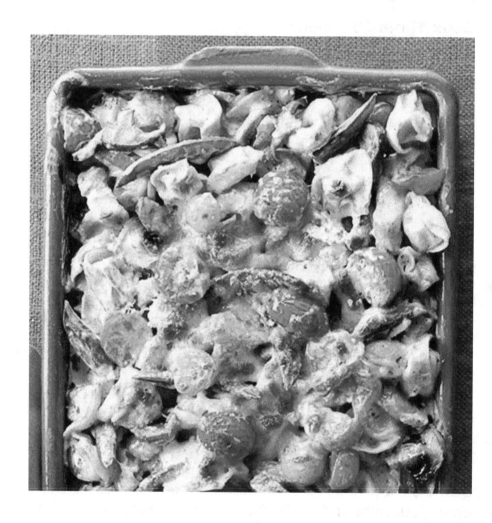

Cod & Veggie Pizza

Prep Time: 20 minutes

Cook Time: 1 hour

Serve: 3

Ingredients:

For Base:

- Olive oil cooking spray
- ¼ cup oat flour
- 2 teaspoons dried rosemary, crushed
- Freshly ground black pepper, to taste
- 4 egg whites
- 2½ teaspoons olive oil
- ½ cup low-fat Parmesan cheese, grated freshly 2 cups zucchini, grated and squeezed

For Topping:

- 1 cup tomato paste
- 1 teaspoon fresh rosemary, minced
- 1 teaspoon fresh basil, minced
- Freshly ground black pepper, to taste
- 4 cups fresh mushrooms, chopped
- 1 tomato, chopped
- 3 ounces boneless cod fillet, chopped
- 1½ cups onion, sliced into rings

- 1 red bell pepper, seeded and chopped
- 1 green bell-pepper, seeded and chopped 1/3 cup low-fat mozzarella, shredded

Instructions:

1.Preheat your oven to 400 degrees F.

2.Grease a pie dish with cooking spray.

3.For base: in a large bowl, add all the ingredients and mix until well combined.

4.Transfer the mixture into prepared pie dish and press to smooth the surface.

5.Bake for approximately 40 minutes.

6. Remove from the oven to cool and set aside for at least 15 minutes.

7.Carefully turn out the crust onto a baking sheet.

8.For topping: in s bowl, add tomato paste, herbs and black pepper.

9.Spread tomato sauce mixture over crust evenly.

10.Arrange the vegetables over tomato sauce, followed by the cheese.

11.Bake for about 21 minutes or until cheese is melted.

Garlicky Haddock

Prep Time: 10 minutes

Cook Time: 11 minutes

Serve: 2

Ingredients:

- 2 tablespoons olive oil, divided
- 4 garlic cloves, minced and divided
- 1 teaspoon fresh ginger, grated finely
- 2 (4-ounce) haddock fillets
- Salt and freshly ground black-pepper, to taste 3 C. fresh baby spinach

Instructions:

1.In a skillet, heat one normal spoon of oil over medium heat and sauté 2 garlic cloves and ginger for about 1 minute.

2.Add the haddock fillets, salt and black pepper and cook for about 3-5 minutes per side or until desired doneness.

3. Meanwhile, heat the remaining oil over medium heat in another skillet, and heat and sauté the remaining garlic for about 1 minute.

4.Ad the spinach, salt and black pepper and cook for about 4-5 minutes.

5.Divide the spinach onto serving plates and top each with 1 haddock fillet.

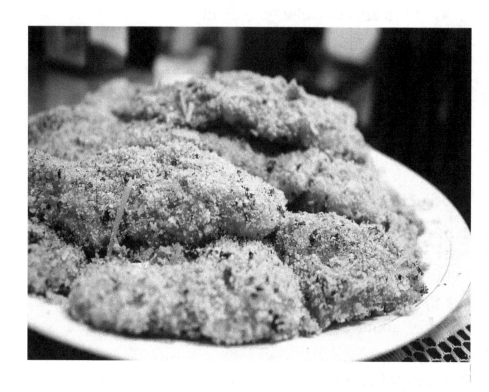

CPSIA information can be obtained
at www.ICGtesting.com
Printed in the USA
LVHW021733010421
683230LV00002B/56